Emily Ryan Investigates

THE SAN ANTONIO MURDER

Mysteries for Seniors

seniorality

The San Antonio Murder - Emily Ryan, Matthew Benson

Copyright © 2024
Seniority / Everbreeze Media Oy

This is a work of fiction. Names and characters are the product of the author's imagination and any resemblance to actual persons, living or dead, is entirely coincidental.

Set in 22 pt EB Garamond

Chapter 1
Checking In

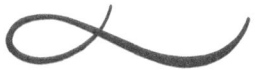

THERE was a cloudless blue sky as I stepped off the final step of the aircraft's exit ramp. I was directed to the interior of the airport to pick up my luggage. I was excited to finally be in San Antonio.

I had heard so much about the city; from its famous canals and architecture, to the remnants of the still-standing Alamo. It was one of Texas' most historical cities, and I was here to bring it to life in the latest issue of LIFE magazine.

As a tenured LIFE journalist, it was my responsibility to photograph and write about all the city's famous landmarks. But first, I would need to get checked into my hotel and set up a base of operations.

The airport workers all wore blue Texas-themed livery, and they were very gracious as they retrieved my large suitcase.

It contained the precious camera that I'd received some years before from my mother as a graduation gift, as well as the computer that I used for writing about the places I visited. It was a huge, bulky contraption and I preferred writing on my typewriter back at the office in New

York, but it did the job while I was out on assignment.

After picking up my luggage, it was time to catch a taxi to my hotel, which I had booked weeks in advance. The agency paid for it - of course.

I stepped back out into the hot summer air and flagged down a bright yellow cab. It wasn't difficult, as there must have been twenty cabs waiting for people to leave the airport. After only a few seconds, one pulled up next to me, and the driver lowered its tinted window.

"Could you take me to the Crockett Hotel?" I asked. "It's on, let me see," I looked at the crinkled piece of paper I'd jotted the address down on earlier, "Bonham Street, that's right."

The taxi driver chuckled. "Yes ma'am, I can get you there. It's a very famous hotel, I'm sure you know, built almost one hundred years ago."

"Oh yes, that's why I chose it. I prefer to stay at the more lived-in places when I'm traveling," I responded.

"Well, I say you've got great taste. The Crockett is a beautiful hotel. Go ahead and hop in the back and I'll get you there in just about twenty minutes," said the driver as he consulted a crumpled old map of the city taped to his dashboard. "This time of day the highway tends to be pretty congested, so we'll take the back roads if necessary."

I grimaced. "I figured. It's about the time everyone gets off work." As the driver lifted my suitcase into the trunk, I climbed into the cab. The inside of the cab was spacious and smelled of bluebonnets- the state flower of Texas.

The seats were clean leather, and the taxi agency had even placed brochures in the pockets behind the front seats. They were full of information about the city. Everything from hotels, restaurants, and tourist destinations was documented. I grabbed one and stuffed it into my purse.

"So, what brings you to San Antonio this fine July?" The driver said as he pulled out of the airport parking lot.

"I'm a journalist with LIFE Magazine. I'm here to photograph the landscape and notable places, then write an article on the city. The last time we had someone down here in San Antonio was thirty years ago and the whole city was colored dark by the Kennedy tragedy in Dallas. The agency would like to see some more light-hearted content for the next edition of our magazine. We're doing an entire issue about America's historic cities."

"Oh, I'm sure. I was only a boy then, but I remember all the adults being quite upset."

"Yes, even back in New York everyone was in mourning. I was on my first assignment as a photographer then and had the hardest time since no one wanted to talk and businesses closed early."

The mood went dark after mention of the Kennedy slaying, and conversation slowed down until the taxi driver, named David, began talking about the places they drove past. Of course, we saw the usual fast food and department stores, but soon enough the taxi began passing more notable locations.

"To your left are the Japanese tea gardens, planted back in 1917, the same year as the Russian Revolution." David's voice began to take on the qualities of a tour guide as we drove through the city outskirts.

"Right next to the gardens is the city zoo. It's been there a little longer, since 1914."

Along the way, they also passed several parks and schools, with which David was less familiar. "To your right is Woody Tucker Park, and it's, well, it's a park," he laughed. As we got downtown the locations became more important.

David's voice became more serious once we drove over the first of many of the city's famous canals. "These are the canals, which I am sure you've heard of. They were originally meant to supply water to the many settlements in the area, including the Alamo, which you will soon see coming up on your left."

Sure enough, it did come up on the left, along with my hotel for the next five days, the Crockett. Its beautiful limestone facade blended in perfectly with the rest of the city. The historical charm and significance were not lost on me and I felt honored to get to stay in the storied city of San Antonio.

David accidentally bumped the dashboard while inputting the mileage for the fare and a radio presenter's voice filled the car. "-in as we progress. The victim, Mr. Bronson, was 30 years old, and was found in his apartment in the city. Police say they do not have a suspect as of-" David cut the radio off.

"I'm so sorry about that, here's your receipt, you have yourself a great stay. I know you'll enjoy the city."

"Oh, of course, yes, and you enjoy the rest of your day, David," I said. I tipped the driver generously and took in the sight of my home for the next five days. The mention of a murder on the radio had caught my attention, and I found it hard to focus on the task at hand.

"Getting into my hotel, that's right," I said out loud. After popping the handle out of my suitcase, I approached The Crockett, pulling the deluxe bag behind me. Two large glass doors opened automatically, and I was greeted by a smiling woman wearing the hotel's uniform.

"Good afternoon, and welcome to The Crockett hotel," the receptionist said. Her name tag read Rachel.

"Good afternoon," I replied. "My name is Emily Ryan. I've got a room booked for the next five days, number 109."

"Room 109, could you please give me your driver's license?" I got the license out of my purse and placed it in Rachel's outstretched hand. The receptionist looked at it funny. "New York huh?" Rachel said, smiling at me.

She scanned it into her computer, then after a few seconds of typing she handed the license back along with a set of keys.

"Here you go. Room 109 is on the second floor. Take the elevator to your left, and your room is the second one on the right. Enjoy your stay," she waved as I began walking towards the elevator.

"Thank you, I will," I called back as I placed my license back into my purse.

Now that I had my room key, I felt like a load had been lifted off my shoulders. I had a place to stay and a job to do. Just how I liked it.

I walked across the wooden floor towards the elevator. The entrances to various historical rooms and shops stood out, but for now, I just wanted to get into my room and shower.

The second floor was much more modern. It had carpeted floors, and each room was guarded by large reinforced doors.

My room was marked by a large metal placard that read '109'. I slid my key into the door and twisted it. Sure enough, the door opened, revealing my room.

Just like the hallway, the room had a plush green carpet filled with spiral patterns. The interior was modern, with drywalls and a ceiling painted beige. The furniture was also modern. A queen-sized bed dominated the room, along with a simple wooden desk. The hotel did have more historic rooms, but they weren't equipped with the amenities that I needed, like electrical outlets.

After a thorough inspection of the room, I began emptying my suitcase. First, I removed the camera and computer, which I placed carefully on the desk. Next, I began removing the clothes I had packed. They went into a small wooden dresser in the room. Finally, I transferred all my toiletries to the bathroom and sat down at the desk.

Work didn't start until tomorrow, so I had the rest of the night to enjoy. The only thing left to do was call my editor and let him know that I had landed safely and had checked into my hotel without any problems.

I used the telephone included in the room to dial his number. Since he was in New York, he was an hour ahead, which is why I needed to call him sooner rather than later.

After a few rings, he picked up. "Good evening, Spielman's office. How can I help you?"

"Hi Francis, it's me, Emily. I made it to San Antonio all right, and I have just checked into my hotel. How are you doing?"

"Oh, hello Emily! I'm glad you made it there in one piece. I was just clocking out for the night. You make sure to be careful and enjoy yourself, you hear?"

I smiled. "I will, Francis. And you be careful too. Good night."

"Goodnight."

Now that I had checked in with my editor, I could go to eat dinner in the city – but, I had the perfect restaurant in mind. The Crockett Tavern was right downstairs and regularly prepared complementary dinners for guests of the hotel.

After showering and getting dressed, I made my way back down to the first floor and headed to the tavern.

The restaurant had a Wild West theme that was used to decorate the whole room. Paintings on the wall depicted the battle for the Alamo and driftwood rafters held hanging saddles and wagon spokes. Old oil lanterns hung near the entrances and exits and the servers all wore old western vests adorned with bandanas and badges.

Everything considered, the place felt very authentic. After being seated, I ordered the restaurant special and waited for my food to arrive. While waiting, I overheard two women discussing details of the murder I had first heard about on the radio.

"They still haven't found the killer," one woman said.

"I know, and it's been almost a week since they broke the news," said the other.

A killer in town? I needed to ask some questions, I thought. It was a bad habit of mine, sticking my nose where it didn't belong.

I approached the table. One of the women had long red hair, and the other short blond hair.

"Excuse me, ladies, were you talking about the recent murder in town?"

"Uh, yes. Who are you?" asked the redhead.

"My name is Emily Ryan. I'm a journalist with LIFE Magazine. I'm not questioning you on official business, I was just interested in the recent murder case."

"The murder... It was last Monday. They said he was killed in his apartment, and the police are still looking for the killer. The victim was some kind of construction worker. They don't even have a suspect though. There's a reward waiting for anyone who saw anything near the scene of the crime."

"A reward, huh? They must be short of leads," I thought to myself.

"Is that all you know?" I asked.

"That's all the information that's publicly available," said the blonde.

"Well, thank you. You two enjoy your dinner." I smiled and went back to my seat and the two women slowly restarted their earlier conversation.

After finishing the dinner I ordered, I went back up to my room and added all the information I'd learned from the two women to my file on San Antonio. It was beginning to look like I might be doing more than taking photos while in the city.

Chapter 2
The Gatekeeper

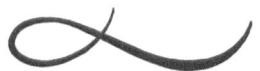

THE NEXT morning, I made sure to get up early. I wanted to be at the front of the line for the Alamo. It was a cool, but humid morning in San Antonio, and the line was not as long as I expected. I was able to finish my visit with the other tourists before seven and had the rest of the morning to kill.

The actual photo-shoot of the Alamo would come later. The agency had organized a date with the local government so I could come while the destination was closed. That way, I could get pictures from all the angles I wanted without there being people in the way.

The Crockett had another in-house restaurant, this one was called the Blue-Jay. It served only breakfast and closed at ten. It was the perfect place to fill up before hitting the city. The interior was very different from the Tavern. Blue-Jay had a strong 1950s theme, and every wall was covered in memorabilia from that decade. Everyone from Elvis to Monroe was represented in the form of novelty plates and knick-knacks.

The place had a lot of the same charm that my parents' kitchen did when I was growing up. Despite all the work that went into making the café look memorable, there weren't a lot of guests. I suppose they're all at the complimentary breakfast, I thought to myself. I ordered the 'Texas Breakfast' - a huge meal consisting of a stack of pancakes drenched in syrup, sausage links, fried eggs, and hash browns. I managed to finish everything except for the pancakes before heading out.

The destination for today was the canals, which were all over the city. I had a few destinations pre-selected, mainly places I already knew were photogenic. For the rest of my photos, I would need to scout around for good vantage points.

I took the bus to my first photo spot, where an unfortunately placed metal railing blocked me from getting the perfect shot. After a few minutes of unsuccessfully repositioning, I was almost ready to give up and head to the next spot when I spotted a police officer.

I approached politely and said, "Good afternoon, officer. Would it be possible for you to unlock the gate to this rail so I could snap a quick photo of the canal?"

"I'm afraid not," replied the officer with a gruff voice. "The rail is there for your safety, and it's only opened for maintenance access."

"Oh well. Sorry for bothering you," I said. I would just have to find another spot for the pictures.

"Wait." It was the officer's voice again. "May I ask why you're taking pictures of the canals?"

"Of course. I'm a photographer for LIFE Magazine and we're doing an article on the city. I need pictures of the canals because they're one of the most famous landmarks here. I wanted to get a closer shot because the canals are probably going to be the background for the cover."

"Really? Could you show me an I.D.? If you're really with LIFE, I might be able to let you through. It's a small world, my daughter actually works there as an intern."

"Sure, here you go." I fished the LIFE lanyard out of my purse and handed it to the officer.

"Let me see..." The officer, whose name tag read Robert, inspected my lanyard. "This looks in order, I think you are who you say you are." He handed the lanyard back. "Let me get the key and I'll open it up for you. Only for a few minutes though."

"Thank you so much," I said. "It really means a lot, and you're helping us get this piece done right. Would you like me to credit you in the article, Robert?"

"No thank you," Robert said forcefully. "I don't need the higher ups knowing that I'm opening the gates for civilians. I'd get written up for sure."

The officer found the key in his squad car nearby. A black metal gate led past the railing and onto the concrete platform directly above the canals. I spent about five minutes taking pictures and had managed to get about ten really good ones that I would be able to present to my editor.

"That's all I needed, Officer, thank you."

"No problem, ma'am," Robert said, quickly closing the gate.

"By the way," I said as I tucked my camera back into my bag. "Do you happen to know anything about the recent murder in the city? I'm not planning on writing about it in our article, I'm just curious."

"Oh yeah, the Branson case. The victim was killed in that apartment building right there." Officer Robert pointed at the towering brick building across the canal. "If I remember right, room 320 is still a crime scene, and I wouldn't advise you to go investigate it for yourself." He looked at the building then back down at Emily. "They're acting really touchy about this case back at the office, the detectives won't really discuss it with us."

Interesting, I thought. I wonder if there's more to the case than meets the eye, or if they're trying to hide their incompetence. Either way, I needed to know more.

"Thank you, Officer Robert. I was just curious, that's all. It's my first time visiting San Antonio and everyone's talking about this murder, so I wanted to know more." I didn't want to raise any suspicion against myself, so I smiled soothingly at the officer.

"Of course, I understand," he replied.

Once Officer Robert had closed the metal gate, we had a conversation about tourism and journalism in the city. We exchanged contact information. As Robert's daughter was a LIFE intern, he thought it would be nice to have a direct link inside the company. After our talk, we parted ways, and I headed back into town for lunch.

The place I had in mind was called 'Three Gringos'. It was a Tex-Mex restaurant that was only open for half of the week. I had needed to reserve a seat ahead of time because it was so popular, and I was excited to learn why.

The restaurant interior was very industrial, with high, unfinished ceilings, and basic stone walls from which an occasional painting or accolade hung.

The staff members were very polite and I ordered today's special, the enchilada platter. The food was good, but not reservation good. In the end, I concluded that the Three Gringos was slightly overrated and I would have to go elsewhere for tomorrow's lunch.

My next goal for the day was to go photograph some of the unspoilt natural areas on the outskirts of the town, but the 'Branson case' as Officer Robert had called it kept eating at me. The apartment where it happened was only a block away, and it certainly wasn't illegal to visit.

I made the walk to the huge brick building and got my LIFE lanyard back out. It gave me an air of authority Hopefully, people would see my ID card and just assume I was someone working for a local news agency.

According to a laminated map on the wall, the room I was looking for was on the third floor. I was relieved to have made it to the elevator with no issues. There were apartments back in New York where you needed a code to get into the main lobby, and I was glad this one wasn't like that.

A shrill ding announced that the elevator had reached the ground floor, and I stepped in and departed for the third floor. It was quiet; no one was walking in the hallway.

The placards on the doors indicated that room 320 was at the end of the hall. I walked silently towards my destination, though I did not creep. It was important to maintain an air of purpose, as it made me seem less suspicious.

A red clip hung from the door handle of room 320. It had white letters and numbers on it, but was unintelligible to me. It probably meant something to the police.

Using the sleeve of my cardigan to prevent the transfer of any fingerprints, I put pressure on the door handle. It moved downwards, meaning that it wasn't locked. This was my chance to learn more. Despite the danger, I simply could not resist a good mystery.

Thankfully, the door was well oiled and opened with no fanfare. The carpeted floor made a crunching sound when I stepped in, which made my heart skip a beat.

"It's just mud," I whispered to myself, looking down.

From the looks of things, the police had already collected their evidence and cleaned up the crime scene, but I took pictures of the entire room, just in case they missed anything.

The only item of note in the room was a packet of papers lying on the victim's desk. After thumbing through them, I had an idea of the victim's employment situation.

It seemed the manager was putting pressure on the victim and his co-workers to resign. The papers did not say why, but they did include the phone numbers and home addresses of several of the people involved, which I quickly wrote down.

Having collected all the evidence there was to be seen in the room, I made my exit. The journey back to the outside world was as easy as the journey in had been.

As soon as I stepped outside, I felt the humid Texas air on my face and I felt the tension leave my shoulders. I had done it. I had collected my evidence and was now ready to start working on the case.

Chapter 3
Seeking Answers

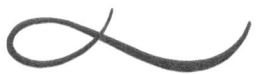

I WAS tired after an afternoon of photographing the unique Spanish architecture of the city. The images would get their own article, written by another LIFE Magazine writer who had more expertise on the subject. The rest of the day was mine alone and I wanted to know more about the Branson case.

I had written down the address of one of the victim's co-workers and a look at a city map revealed that he lived not far from where I was. It would certainly help advance my case if I could question him before dinner. Just like lunch, I had reservations at a fancy restaurant in town, and could not be late. The questioning would have to be brief.

The co-worker was named Maxwell Graham according to the file. He lived in a suburb a few miles away from downtown, so I took a bus and walked the rest of the way.

The neighborhood was nice. Freshly cut grass and clean side walks showed that the people who lived here cared about their environment and how it reflected on them.

Maxwell's house was no different to any of the others on his street. It was built in the Texas Ranch style, and featured a huge framed window looking into the kitchen and dining area. I knocked on the door three times and waited. A pickup truck was parked in the driveway, so I assumed he was home.

Just as I was about to turn around and give up for the day, I heard the door unlock, then crack open.

"Hello?" A man's voice said.

"Hello. Are you Maxwell Graham?" I replied.

"Uh, yes. Who am I speaking to?" He still hadn't opened the door any further.

"My name is Emily, and I'm a reporter with The New York Times." A white lie. I used to work for the NYT when I was younger, and LIFE didn't really cover murders.

If Maxwell was intelligent enough to know that, then he'd be suspicious of me, and I didn't want that. "I wanted to ask you a few questions about the passing of your co-worker, Charlie Branson." I tried tilting my head to get a better view inside, but the door was basically still shut.

"Why should I speak to you? Reporters are nothing but trouble," he grumbled.

"Wait! Before you close the door, just listen. I'm not here on official business, just looking into this for myself. I won't publish anything that you say, I only want to know what happened that day."

The door opened a little wider and Maxwell eyed me suspiciously. "I'll give you five minutes." He finally opened the door all the way and stepped outside. "Ask."

"Thank you. What was the atmosphere on the job site like on the days before the murder? Did anyone act differently, or was there tension between the employees that wasn't there before?"

"No, we all did our jobs as usual. There was no theatrics. The only one acting differently was that damn manager. Corporate is constantly breathing down his neck to increase margins and he's taken that to mean forcing us to quit."

"He was forcing you to quit? What do you mean?" I asked.

"It's exactly as it sounds. He was pressuring ten percent of the laborers to resign, so he could get the budget where he needed it to be. He's been a bundle of stress for the last few weeks, a nightmare to deal with."

"Hmm, and was he-"

"It's been five minutes, times up." Maxwell cruelly smiled and slammed the door shut.

"So much for that. What a rude man," I muttered to myself.

He was my only lead at the moment and his unwillingness to talk made him suspicious. The manager's behavior was out of place too. I would need to pay him a visit as well.

Luckily his information had also been inside that packet of papers I found in the victim's apartment, though he lived further into the suburbs than Maxwell. I would have to take the bus again, but for now I needed to get back to my hotel and prepare for dinner.

The ride back was uneventful and I had plenty of time to think about my next move.

As for motive, it was likely one of his co-workers had killed him. There was competition to see who would get to stay on in the job, and the manager was putting pressure on them all. It's easy to understand a man with a family thinking he needs the money much more than a single man.

Back at the hotel I showered and got dressed for the night. The restaurant I was going to tonight was called 'Eduardo's'. It supposedly started out as a Mexican restaurant then transformed into a three-star Michelin destination.

The meal was uneventful. Just like The Three Gringos, Eduardo's was overrated. It seemed like the food scene in San Antonio just didn't compare to New York. I decided to stick to The Crockett's in-house restaurants for the rest of the trip. The food was good and wasn't overpriced, nor did you have to dress up to eat.

The next day I headed straight to the job site. The packet that I got my information from had not included the manager's schedule, so I didn't want to get there after he'd already left. The job site was loud. The sound of jackhammers pounding into the earth and the scream of diesel engines filled the air.

According to a sign at the entrance, they was construction work on a new apartment building, since San Antonio's population was constantly growing and needed new housing. So far they had the foundation done and were installing the metal frame of the first floor.

The manager's office was inside a portable trailer. He wasn't the highest ranking person related to the project, but he was the only high ranking individual that was actually on site every day. That made him the most important person in the eyes of the workers.

I knocked on his door, hopeful that I had made it in time to catch him. The door was flimsy plastic and had a significant give when I pressed on it. After only a few seconds, the door opened, revealing a very sweaty middle-aged man wearing a white button-up and dress pants. He frowned slightly when he saw me. He was most likely expecting one of his workers.

"Hello, how can I help you, ma'am?"

"Hello, my name is Emily, and I'm an investigative journalist. I wanted to ask you some questions about the recent passing of an employee of yours."

"Oh, that. Um, well, go ahead and come in. I have a little time and can answer some of your questions." He turned around and gestured for me to follow him in.

The carpet inside the trailer was crunchy with dried mud, and old fast food wrappers were piled up in a plastic trash can that should have been taken out weeks ago.

"Welcome, my name is Michael, by the way. What did you need to know?" He sat down behind his desk in a tall office chair, and I sat down in a plush guest chair, facing him.

"Could you tell me about the victim? What was Mr. Branson like? Did he like to tell jokes, or was he a more reserved man?"

"He was, how should I say? He was a very matter-of-fact man. He came to work every day on time, did the bare minimum, and left. He never made friends with anyone, nor caused any problems. I would've described him as a real loner."

"A loner? Okay, thank you. What about his private life? In your time knowing him, did he reveal anything about himself?"

"No, he never spoke about himself. Aside from when I first interviewed him, he only spoke about his previous experience doing construction work. He said that he'd worked across the country, and his record was legit."

"Interesting. So you don't know anything about his personal life?"

"No and not for lack of trying. After his tragic passing, I went through his record looking for a parent or relative to contact and found nothing. Even the emergency phone number he gave us didn't answer. I'm sure the police know more about him; he kept his work life and private life completely separate."

"Thank you. And what about his co-workers? Did any of them have a negative opinion of him?"

"Not exactly. While he didn't create problems with anyone, he was distant. There are guys on the team that react negatively to quiet, unresponsive men. I guess because they don't get help inflating their ego, they see them as trying to undermine them in some way."

He continued, "There was a guy, Maxwell, who was constantly telling jokes and riling the other guys up. Branson didn't participate, which offended Maxwell. Nothing really came of it, but I went ahead and assigned them to different areas on the site, just to be careful."

So, he was hiding something from me, I thought as that is certainly useful information.

"Did you happen to-" I was interrupted by an alarm going off in the office.

Michael jumped up and said, "I'm so sorry, but that's the fume alarm. We've got an old jack hammer that sometimes smokes up. I have to go make sure they turn it off."

He pulled on a thick black overcoat and ran outside, yelling something that I couldn't hear.

I decided to seize on the opportunity and document the manager's office.

Starting off with his desk, he had a stack of Employee files. I photographed the one on top and looked over a few others. There didn't seem to be any relevant information.

Next, I combed through some of the documents that pertained to the project's budget and got confirmation that the manager was being pressured to decrease his workforce.

Listed in the details of one document were the specifics of the severance packages and they seemed quite generous. I wondered why none of the employees so far had accepted the offer.

After photographing the rest of the office, I exited the trailer and went looking for someone that I could question. Someone on break would be perfect.

In the end, I had only managed to find one worker who wasn't busy, and he didn't have much to say. Only that so far no one had decided to leave.

When I asked him about the severance package, he looked at me funny. Before

I could question him any more, his co-workers began calling his name and he jogged off.

It was now slightly past midday, and I wanted to question Maxwell again– the rude man I had first spoken to at this apartment - as the manager, Michael, had said incriminating things about him.

He was off work today, so I would have to visit his home once more. I took the same bus as last time and made my way through the winding streets of Maxwell's neighborhood.

I began to hear sirens as I got closer to his house, and once I reached his street, I saw the blue and red flashing lights indicative of emergency vehicles. There was an army of police and firemen outside the house that I visited yesterday.

I approached one of the officers on the outskirts of the scene and asked him what had happened.

"Some kind of attack. The victim was taken to the hospital. That's all I can say."

The police wouldn't allow me access, so I had no choice but to go back to my hotel for the day. I was sitting on my bed, eating lunch and watching T.V. when the local news broadcaster announced that there had been another murder in the city. This time it was the man I spoke to yesterday - Maxwell Hurst.

Chapter 4
Unravelling Motives

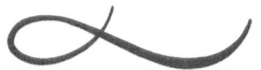

I FELT a bit down after the news. Murder is generally a good cause for sadness, but I was also upset about my case. Maxwell had gone from prime suspect to innocent victim in one day.

I had been totally off regarding Branson's murder and was going to have to start over from zero if I wanted to solve the case.

Later that night, after I had eaten dinner and showered, I got a call from my editor, Francis.

"Hello, this is Emily Ryan speaking."

"Good evening, Emily. This is Francis. Just checking in on you. How goes the photo shoot?"

"It's going quite well. I have almost everything I need, and I've got lots of good stuff to write about. How are you doing?"

"Eh, I'm okay. A couple of people at our office got laid off. Budget cuts is what my boss said. It's got everyone in a sour mood."

"Aah, I'm sorry to hear that, Francis", I replied. Budget cuts huh, I thought to myself. Sounds like they're going through something similar to what I'm dealing with.

"Don't worry about it" assured Francis. "Our team got off scot-free. They're really happy with the work we're doing, actually".

"Well, I'm glad to hear that at least," I sighed. After Maxwell's death, I wondered if the budget cuts were still a part of the motive?

"Are you really doing okay? You sound upset?"

"I'm fine. It's just…"

"You picked up another case again, didn't you?"

"You know me so well. I've come up against a brick wall, and don't see any way forward. I thought I was doing so well, too."

"Ha-ha. That just proves that you're a journalist, not a detective. Leave that work to the police and save yourself the trouble."

"You know, you're right. I think I will," I said with a smile.

"You're a horrible liar."

My smile turned to laughter. "Have a good night, Francis."

"You, too."

The next morning I ate breakfast at the hotel's café. Afterwards, I left to do the final photo shoot for San Antonio. Since I had already captured the most notable things about the city, today was a day for me to leisurely walk around and photograph whatever stood out to me and captured the character of the city.

In some kind of providential coincidence, I came across one of the workers I saw on the job site yesterday. He looked like he was with his son. When the boy ran off to buy something from a food truck, I took the chance to go and talk to him.

"Hey, you work under Michael Johnson, at the construction site a few miles from here, right?"

"Uh, yes. Do I know you?"

"Probably not. I'm the wife of one of your co-workers. I was wondering why none of you had taken the severance package yet? I know Michael wants some of you gone and the deal seems pretty sweet to me. What gives?"

"What severance? He wants us to quit, there's no clause that says we get anything after we quit."

"Wait, it's not a lay-off deal?" I asked.

"Hell no. If it was, I'm sure someone would have accepted by now. We don't get anything out of quitting. We all figured between ourselves that we should stay no matter what. That way we'd be forcing that nasty manager to either lay us off or fire us, in which we would be able to claim unemployment." He sounded angry as he spoke.

The little boy was running back with a hot dog.

"Thank you, I need to go check something," I said, making my excuses.

I raced back to my hotel to check my photos. If what he said was true, then the manager just became the number one suspect in my case.

Sure enough, one of the photos I had taken revealed a packet of papers detailing the severance benefits.

I had taken the photo before I originally went through the papers and it looked almost like it was hidden, stuffed underneath a bunch of employee files.

"This is great news," I thought. "I need to bring this to the attention of the police." I dialed the number of Officer Robert. It rang eight times then went to voicemail. I called again, and he picked up after three rings.

"Hello, is this Officer Robert, with the San Antonio police?"

"Yes it is. Who am I speaking with?" replied the voice I recognized.

"Oh, it's great to hear your voice, Robert. This is Emily Ryan, the LIFE journalist. We met a few days ago. You did me a favor at the canals."

"Oh Emily, how's it going?" Officer Robert asked, greeting her warmly.

"I'm well, but I've got an important update in the Branson case."

The officer didn't respond, so I kept going.

"I've discovered that the victim's manager, Michael, is pressuring his employees to quit and hiding the fact that they will receive severance pay if they get laid off instead. Originally, I thought the motive was employee competition. One employee killing others to secure his position, but I've changed my mind." I said, pausing for effect.

"I believe the manager has a stronger motive since he is likely to be in a position to lose his job if he doesn't decrease his workforce. He's killing his own employees to save himself from having to fire them or lay them off. That way there's no severance pay - or unemployment."

"Emily, I thought you were a LIFE reporter. LIFE reporters don't investigate murders, they take pictures and write articles. Why are you sticking your nose into this? I thought I told you to leave it alone." Robert sounded suddenly annoyed.

"I'm sorry, but I believe I know who the killer is and there's no one else for me to tell. Please tell me that you guys are at least considering him as a suspect."

"I wouldn't be able to tell you even if I knew. We're accepting anonymous tips from people who were near the scene of the crime, but not unsolicited investigation advice."

I was growing frustrated. "Okay, but where can I-" the call ended abruptly.

"Dang it," Emily exclaimed out loud.

I was unsure what I should do next. He sounded confident that they didn't need my input, so maybe I should have just left it to them, but I wasn't convinced.

I spent the rest of the day photographing the city, but I couldn't get the case out of my mind.

After eating dinner and getting ready for bed, I couldn't help myself from going over all the photos I had assembled for my case. One in particular stood out to me. It was the photo I had taken of the manager's desk.

The manager had been going through a stack of employee files and the one on top of the pile caught my eye. It was for a Mr. Chad Berg.

I began to worry that he might be the manager's next target. If he really was the murderer, then this was the last employee that he had looked into, making him the next most likely target.

There was nothing I could do though. I had already alerted the police and they weren't receptive. The best I could do was hope that they took their jobs seriously. That night I went to bed full of worry and doubt and had a dreamless and restless sleep.

Chapter 5
An Anxious Wait

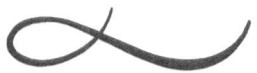

I SPENT the next day out in town, trying to distract myself from the murder case. The last thing I wanted to see or hear was another reported killing.

I had already taken all the photos I needed of the city and had finished the first draft of my article.

Tomorrow would be my last day in San Antonio and I wanted to enjoy the city while not working. Not that I didn't enjoy my job. I liked working, but I also enjoyed the feeling of having my responsibilities behind me - especially in a big city, where there was so much to do and explore.

After a quick brunch at a nice little Italian-themed café, I went back to the Alamo - as a tourist. I had visited twice before. Once for pictures and once in passing.

This time I was a part of an official tour group and got to enjoy the guide's many stories and history lessons about the old Spanish fort.

The tour guide's speech conjured visions of groups of men fighting to death for what they believed in. It was a powerful image and it caused me to reconsider my abandonment of the Branson case.

I imagined myself being possessed by the spirit of one of those brave men, and going to apprehend the suspect despite not having any police support. It was a fantasy of course. Even if I could overpower the manager, I had no legal authority to do anything. I'd be the one breaking the law.

There really was nothing I could do without the police. My one contact inside the force had treated me nicely at first, but had turned surprisingly cold.

I suspected that it was because of department politics. Higher-ups were likely upset at the way the case was going and taking it out on the people lower in the hierarchy. That's why the case was a sore spot for Officer Robert. It could also be the bureaucracy involved with policing a big city. Being from New York, I was very familiar with the muddled communication and feelings of isolation between different sections of the police.

After the Alamo, I went on a boat tour of the canals. I and a few other tourists got to explore San Antonio from the water and it provided an interesting new perspective.

The lights of the city reflected off of the water and moved with a life of their own. From street level, this phenomenon didn't look nearly as beautiful.

Perspective was important. I would not have originally suspected the manager without the perspective provided by one of the workers.

I thought about the settlers who had originally dug the canals. For them, the work was a matter of life and death and some people had died during their construction. They needed the water for irrigation and hydration, so they dug - no matter the cost.

If the Alamo taught the value of persistence in the face of defeat, the canals taught the value of finishing the job no matter what, because it simply needed to be done.

After my adventure in the canals, I walked through the city one last time. My final day would be mostly spent finishing the final draft of my article. San Antonio was quite charming, even if it was very different from my home, New York.

The beautiful Spanish architecture was definitely something I didn't have back home and the idea that a city so far west could still have old-world charm fascinated me. It made sense, of course. The Spanish had lived here and built in the Spanish style. In my experience, the further west I went, the more modern and American things usually became.

I heard an unfamiliar voice call my name when I was walking back to my hotel for the night. I turned around and saw a man waving me down. He didn't seem threatening, so I stopped and waited for him to catch up to me.

"Hey, Emily. I didn't think I'd see you here," the man said, having caught up to me.

"Um, hello." He looked vaguely familiar. "Do I know you?" I asked.

"Ha ha, I wasn't sure if you'd recognize me. I'm David, your taxi driver from earlier this week."

"Oh, yes it's you." I said with a smile. "I'm sorry I didn't recognize you. I've had a lot on my mind recently."

"Hmm, want to talk about it?" David asked.

"Sure. I'm sure I told you that I'm a journalist, here taking pictures in the city".

"Mmm."

"Well, I don't know why, maybe because I used to be a war journalist, but I've always been drawn to more intense cases". I added. " I took this job because I like living a quiet life, mostly. But every now and then I get the itch to solve an important case. That's what's going on. The murders that have happened in the city recently, I've been looking into them."

David looked shocked and very sceptical. "Really?" He asked.

"Yeah. I think I've solved the case, in fact. I called the police to let them know, and they dismissed me. I know they don't have to listen to me, and that it isn't my responsibility to bring people to justice, I just take pictures, and write about those pictures. But I've got a solid case and can't sleep at night knowing that there's a murder that I could prevent."

"Wait, you think you know the next victim?"

"Yes. I'm certain it's the victims' manager targeting employees that he wants off the job. Corporate is putting pressure on him to reduce costs and he's going about it by forcing his men to quit - without severance."

I paused as I took a deep breath. "I interviewed him a few days ago, and he seemed pleasant, if a little unhygienic. I saw the files of the employees laid out on his desk, and he was looking at one in particular – the one on José Mendez. I believe that he's the next victim."

David was still looking at me inquisitively.

"I know that's only motive and opportunity, but I also discovered physical evidence. I was only able to investigate the first crime scene. One thing that stood out to me was the carpet. It was crunchy with dried mud. It had rained the day before the first murder and at first I figured that it was just from the victim's boots if he came home late."

"I rethought this, however, when I visited the manager and noticed that his carpet was just as dirty. Those two things are not directly linked, but it did make me think. I checked the history of the local weather forecast and compared it to the victim's schedule. He realistically should have been home and sleeping before the rain began. It's possible that the tracks came from the manager sneaking in during the night, while the victim was asleep."

"Hmm, that is suspicious."

"Yeah, I know it's not enough for a conviction outright, but if the police search his home and workspace I'm sure they'll find something. I just wish they'd listen to me."

David was quiet for a minute while we walked. "I might be able to help you," he finally said.

I frowned. "How could you help me?"

David hesitated. "I've got a relative in the police. I could contact him and he could potentially investigate what you've been talking about."

"Really?" I stopped walking and faced David. Do you think it would work? I already reached out to my contact, and he gave me the cold shoulder."

"Yeah." David smiled. "He's actually my brother, and he owes me a favor."

After David got off the phone with his brother, we spent the rest of the evening walking around the city and talking about all the things I had seen and done during my stay. I felt an exciting anxiety, waiting on the result of the investigation. It likely wouldn't come until the next day, however.

After David walked me back to the hotel, the two of us said our goodbyes and I settled in to go to sleep. I stayed up late that night though, watching the news hawkishly, hoping to see the manager's mugshot flash onto the screen.

Chapter 6
Solving the Case

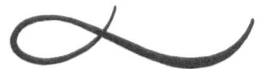

I AWOKE the next morning having only slept for a few hours. The news was still playing on the T.V, but they were doing a segment on a local restaurant and not talking about the murder.

I rolled out of bed and checked my voicemail before beginning my morning routine. Nothing so far. If the police had caught the manager they hadn't released the news yet.

Since today was my last day in the city there wasn't much to do other than pack and make sure both my photographs and writings were in good shape.

I spent the rest of the morning getting my work organized and packing my clothes and toiletries. The local news still played loudly in the background, and I kept my ear open for any mention of a police apprehension.

Once I had finished packing I still had nearly nine hours until I needed to be at the airport. I wasn't sure what to do with the free time. My legs were tired from walking last night, and I had already visited everywhere in the city that I was interested in. Just as I was getting up to go down to the lobby the T.V went silent.

I glanced at it. The screen was dark with no sound for a few seconds and then it cut to a breaking news report.

"Police have apprehended a man who they say is a prime suspect in the Branson murder case, which has had San Antonions on edge this last week," a female announcer said. Images were shown of the police escorting a man with a blurred face into a jail house.

The report went on to summarize the case so far, which I was already familiar with. The man in the photos had the build of manager Michael, but I wasn't sure because his face was blurred.

I needed to call David to confirm, but just as I was about to call, my own phone rang.

"Emily Ryan speaking."

"Emily! Hey, it's David. My brother just called and let me know that they've arrested someone. He can't legally tell me who, but this is coming right after our phone call where I told him about your manager, so it's safe to assume it's him."

"I know, I'm watching the news right now. I can't believe they arrested him though. Shouldn't they bring him in for questioning first?"

"Normally yes. But it's possible that they caught him in the act or maybe he even fought back. Either way they got him, that's cause to celebrate, eh?" David asked.

"Yes. I think it is," I responded. "How about we meet for brunch at the Blue-Jay cafe. Do you know where that is?"

David laughed. "I'm a taxi driver. I know where everything is in this city ."

We met about an hour later at the cafe. David wore a tan cardigan and blue jeans. Today was one of the rare days that it wasn't hot and he had dressed accordingly. To me the weather was still rather warm, so I hadn't layered up any more than I had previously.

We ate our brunch, consisting of coffee, croissants, and fruit bowls while discussing the capture of Michael, the construction site manager.

The cafe had a T.V. on one of its walls and we made sure to grab seats that faced it. Thankfully it played the news 24/7, so we would be able to see any updates on the arrest.

Unfortunately, nothing interesting came on the T.V. and our brunch ended without any updates on the arrest. I do, however, know a lot more about David now and I feel as though I've made a new close friend. If I'm ever back in the city, I'll need to meet with him.

David walked me back to the hotel where I made sure everything was packed for my flight. While I was going through the pictures I had taken, the T.V. in my room cut from an advertisement for medicine to breaking news about the murder.

"This news is just in, police have revealed the identity of their prime suspect in the murder of Richard Branson," the news anchor announced.

The manager's mugshot appeared on the screen. He looked rough. I had seen him in his office, on his territory. Despite the general filth, he had looked calm and behaved very courteously towards me. In the picture, he looked nothing like that. His facial hair was unkempt, and the white shirt and red tie that he wore were torn up.

"Authorities say that the suspect, identified as Michael Bernstein, aged 44 years old, was captured at the residence of what they believe was his next victim."

"Oh my," I thought out loud.

The video cut from the news reporter to a police press conference. Men in police uniforms and suits crowded around the San Antonio chief of police.

"Michael Bernstein was arrested this morning, at 02:42. Officers responded to an anonymous tip off that he might be targeting his own employees. Officers searched the suspect's own residence, finding several pieces of evidence, but not Mr. Bernstein. Officers then made their way to the potential victim's residence, where Mr. Bernstein's vehicle was parked outside."

The chief cleared his throat and continued. "One officer stayed behind at the vehicle and the others went to search for Mr. Bernstein. They ultimately found him in the lobby of the apartment complex where the potential victim lives. He had not yet made it to the victim's apartment, thankfully. Bernstein tried to flee when officers approached, and a small scuffle ensued. At the very least, Mr. Bernstein will be charged with assaulting a police officer, but we are of course investigating his involvement in the recent murderers."

He looked up from the podium and at the audience. "We'll be taking questions now, for the next thirty minutes."

A journalist in the crowd yelled, "Why did it take so long to catch the killer? Do you have any idea about his motive?"

"We originally had no solid suspect. The first victim's family lived out of state and he had almost no friends or acquaintances. That left only his co-workers, and we could not attach a motive to any of them. They also all had solid alibis - Mr. Bernstein included. The nature of what he told the police originally will be revealed in court, but it did lead us to believe at that stage, that he was not a suspect."

The crowd murmured after the mention of court. "As for the motive we have now, it appears to be workplace mismanagement. The company that all the parties work for- Chamberlain Construction- had been pressurizing

Mr. Bernstein to reduce his workforce without directly letting anyone go. This caused him to act out of desperation, eliminating his own employees in order to keep his job."

The press conference went on, with the chief revealing information when he could. Almost everything he said I already knew. It felt good that my information had solved the case, even if I got no credit. The knowledge that I was responsible for the killer's capture was enough.

At the end of the conference, they revealed there would be a memorial for the two victims and their families, which was a nice gesture. The company in charge of the building project had also had its license revoked by the city and was under investigation for violation of labor laws. The project was being taken over by another company and the workers who were out of work would be compensated.

I had to turn my attention away from the T.V. and back to the task at hand. My room was completely packed up, and all the dirty sheets and pillowcases were sitting on the bed ready for housekeeping. It was time to go.

David personally drove me to the airport in his own car. We said our goodbyes and I boarded the plane back to New York.

All things considered, it was a very successful trip. Another mystery solved and another part of the world added to my portfolio. I had taken some incredible photos of San Antonio and the article was going to be a hit. I couldn't wait to show them - along with my written work- to my editor.

Epilogue

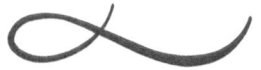

TEN DAYS later, I was sitting in my apartment overlooking Central Park in New York when a news broadcast came on the T.V. It was about the San Antonio murders.

They were doing a memorial for the victims as a part of the San Antonio Riverwalk Parade. It involved huge posters decorated by school children being hoisted high in the air by people standing atop moving floats. It was a beautiful way to remember the victims.

After the parade coverage, my phone rang.

"Emily Ryan speaking."

"Hey Emily, it's Francis. I just wanted to let you know that corporate approved your article. They loved the photos and even commented that this might be your best writing yet."

"That's great to hear, Francis. Any idea when the article will get published?" I asked.

"Ha ha, no idea. It could be next week, or next year. You know how they are."

I smiled. "Yeah, I do."

The End

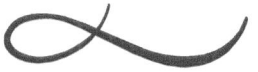

Other Books from Seniorality

To find your next book Emily Ryan book visit:

www.amazon.com/author/seniorality

Where you will find:

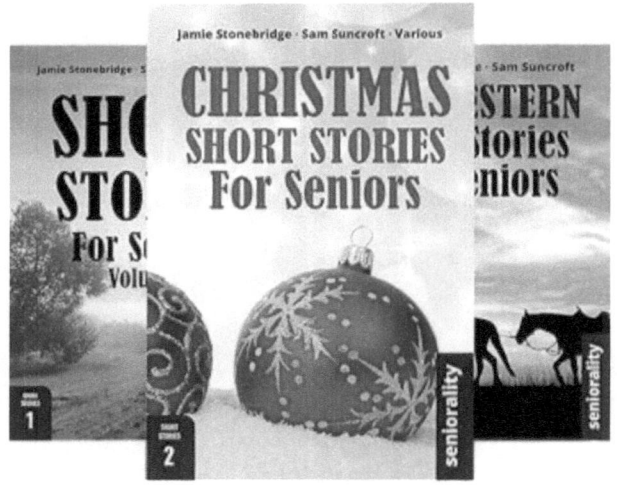

Short Stories

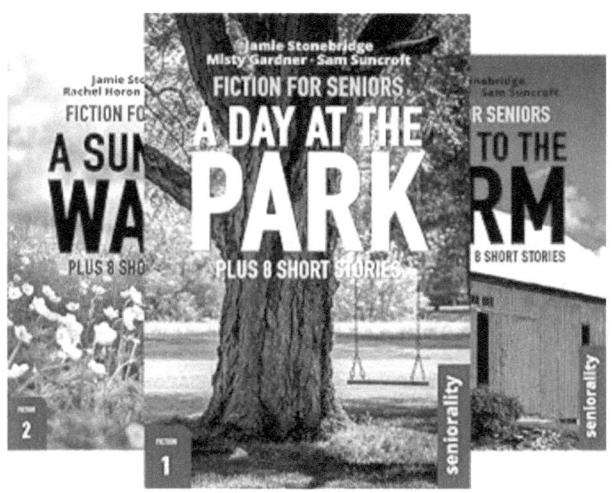

Fiction for Seniors

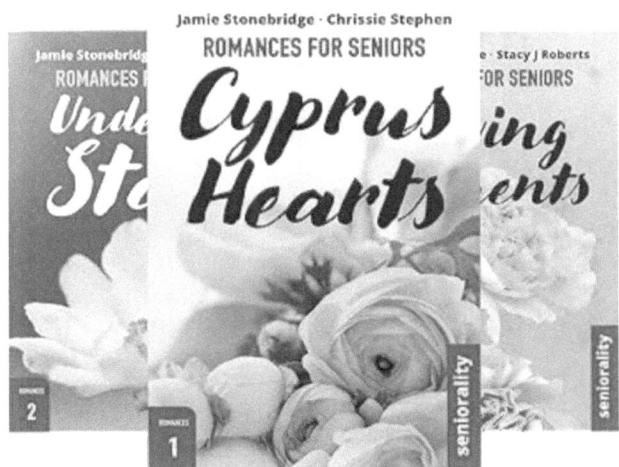

Romances for Seniors

Find these and many more books
by searching on Amazon for 'seniorality'
or visit: **www.amazon.com/author/seniorality**

Thank You

If you enjoyed this book or found it useful, we'd be very grateful if you'd post a short review on Amazon. Your support really does make a difference and helps other people discover this book.

We read all the reviews personally so we can get your feedback to make ours books even better or get ideas for future books.

Thank you and have a wonderful day!

www.ingramcontent.com/pod-product-compliance
Lightning Source LLC
Chambersburg PA
CBHW020442220526
45464CB00002B/820